THE ANTI-INFLAMMATORY VASCULITIS DIET COOKBOOK FOR BEGINNERS

Delightful Homemade DIY Recipes for Eliminating Inflammation, Fortifying Immunity, Preventing Heart Disease, and Achieving Vibrant Health

CAROLINE SIMMONS, MD

Copyright Page

Copyright © 2024 by Caroline Simmons, MD.

The recipes and suggestions provided in this book are for informational purposes only. The author and publisher are not responsible for any adverse effects or consequences resulting from the use of the recipes, dietary practices, or suggestions described herein. Always consult a professional or medical expert if you have any concerns regarding your dietary needs and health conditions.

Table of Contents

1

UNDERSTANDING VASCULITIS

Vasculitis is a condition that causes inflammation (swelling) in your blood vessels.

Blood vessels are channels that carry blood throughout your body. They form a circuit that begins and ends at your heart. You have three types of blood vessels:

Arteries: Arteries carry blood away from your heart to the rest of your body.

Veins: Veins carry blood back to your heart.

Capillaries: Capillaries are small blood vessels that connect your arteries and veins together. If you think about your circulatory system like a network of highways, capillaries are the on-ramps and exits that help your blood move along its route from your heart through your body and back.

If you have vasculitis, your blood vessels swell and thicken. This makes it harder for blood to flow through them. Over time, the inflammation can damage your organs and cause serious complications like aneurysms.

Most people with vasculitis can manage their symptoms with medication. But vasculitis can be fatal if you experience severe symptoms that affect blood flow to your organs.

Visit a healthcare provider if you experience symptoms like fever or feel numbness or tingling in your hands or feet. Call 911 (or your local emergency number) or go to the emergency room if you're having trouble breathing or experiencing heart attack symptoms.

How does vasculitis affect my body?

Vasculitis can affect any blood vessel in your body, including the ones that are connected to your:

Skin.

Lungs.

Heart.

Nerves.

Eyes.

Kidneys.

Brain.

Sinuses.

Stomach.

Hands and feet.

How common is vasculitis?

Vasculitis is rare. Experts estimate fewer than 50 out of every million people in the U.S. develop it each year.

People older than 50 are more likely to develop vasculitis, but it's still rare. Experts estimate that fewer than 300 people in one million people older than 50 in the U.S. are diagnosed with vasculitis each year.

Vasculitis Causes

Doctors don't know exactly what causes many cases of vasculitis. But there are some possible triggers:

Autoimmune diseases like RA, lupus, or Sjögren's syndrome

Infections, such as hepatitis B and hepatitis C, that set off an unusual immune system reaction that damages your blood vessels

Allergic reactions to medications

Certain blood cancers, like leukemia and lymphoma

Risk factors

Vasculitis can happen to anyone. Factors that may increase the risk of certain disorders include:

Age: Giant cell arteritis rarely occurs before the age of 50, while Kawasaki disease is most common in children younger than 5 years old.

Family history: Behcet's disease, granulomatosis with polyangiitis and Kawasaki disease sometimes run in families.

Lifestyle choices: Using cocaine can increase your risk of developing vasculitis. Smoking tobacco, especially if you're a man younger than 45, can increase your risk of Buerger's disease.

Medications: Vasculitis can sometimes be triggered by medications such as hydralazine, allopurinol, minocycline and propylthiouracil.

Infections: Having hepatitis B or C can increase your risk of vasculitis.

Immune disorders: People who have disorders in which their immune systems mistakenly attack their own bodies may be at higher risk of vasculitis. Examples include lupus, rheumatoid arthritis and scleroderma.

Sex: Giant cell arteritis is much more common in women, while Buerger's disease is more common in men.

Overview of Vasculitis Types

Vasculitis is the general term for several conditions that cause blood vessel inflammation. Doctors organize vasculitis into types based on the size of the blood vessels involved. All types of vasculitis can affect anyone, but some are more common in certain age groups.

Systemic vasculitis is inflammation of your blood vessel walls, which can happen anywhere in your body.

Exercise-induced vasculitis is a type of small-vessel vasculitis. It restricts vessels in your lower legs after you do intense exercise like running or hiking, particularly in hot weather. Women over 50 get it most often. Symptoms include rashes on your legs that go away in a few days.

Urticarial vasculitis affects your skin's small blood vessels. The inflammation usually causes patches and hives that can itch, burn, and discolor your skin. If it gets more serious, it may damage other organs, too.

Leukocytoclastic vasculitis results when waste from immune cells in the walls of your small blood vessels causes inflammation. When the damaged blood vessels become leaky, they cause raised spots on your skin, usually your legs. Most of the time, it affects only your skin. But it can spread to other organs if it's serious.

ANCA vasculitis targets a certain type of white blood cell in your body and tells these cells to attack small blood vessels. When the blood vessels are invaded, they become swollen and inflamed. ANCA vasculitis can happen in many parts of your body. The inflammation causes different symptoms, depending on where it is.

IGA vasculitis is the most common type of vasculitis in children. It causes inflammation and bleeding of small blood vessels in your skin, joints, intestines, and kidneys. The most common symptom is a raised skin rash, usually on your legs or buttocks that looks like bruises. But if IGA vasculitis affects other organs, you could have stomach or joint pain, swelling, and kidney inflammation.

Cutaneous vasculitis is when you have inflammation and damage to your skin's blood vessels. It's the most common vasculitis doctors see. It shows up as raised patches on your skin.

Central nervous system (CNS) vasculitis happens when the blood vessel walls in your brain and spine become inflamed. Many conditions can cause it, though your immune system often plays a role. While it's one of the more serious types of vasculitis, it is treatable.

Rheumatoid vasculitis is a complication of rheumatoid arthritis (RA) that happens when the inflammation that causes joint pain and damage also damages your blood vessels. Rheumatoid vasculitis causes your small- and medium-sized blood vessels to become inflamed and narrow. It most often shows up in skin, nerves, fingers, and toes.

Other types of vasculitis include giant cell arteritis, polyarteritis nodosa, Takayasu arteritis, Behçet's disease, and Kawasaki disease.

Complications

Vasculitis complications depend on the type and severity of your condition. Or they may be related to side effects of the prescription medications you use to treat the condition. Complications of vasculitis include:

Organ damage: Some types of vasculitis can be severe, causing damage to major organs.

Blood clots and aneurysms: A blood clot may form in a blood vessel, obstructing blood flow. Rarely, vasculitis will cause a blood vessel to weaken and bulge, forming an aneurysm (AN-yoo-riz-um).

Vision loss or blindness: This is a possible complication of untreated giant cell arteritis.

Infections: Some of the medications used to treat vasculitis may weaken your immune system. This can make you more prone to infections.

Symptoms and Diagnosis

Vasculitis Symptoms

Vasculitis symptoms can show up in many ways, depending on what part of your body is affected. Still, some general symptoms include:

Fever

Weight loss

Loss of appetite

Fatigue

Headache

General aches and pains

Symptoms related to specific areas of your body include:

Eyes: Your first sign of vasculitis might be red, itchy, or burning eyes. You could also see double and have temporary or permanent blindness in one or both eyes.

Skin: You might get rashes, lumps, or open sores if vasculitis affects blood vessels going to your skin.

Nerves: If your nerves don't get enough blood, you could feel numbness, tingling, pain, and weakness.

Brain: Vasculitis in your brain may cause a stroke.

Heart: You could have heart palpitations or even a heart attack if it affects your heart.

Kidneys: Inflammation in the vessels that supply blood to your kidneys can lead to kidney failure.

Digestive system: You may feel pain after you eat if vasculitis affects your stomach or intestines. You could also see blood in your stool.

Ears: Vasculitis can cause your ears to ring. It could also cause dizziness or sudden loss of hearing. You might also get inner ear infections.

Hands and feet: Vasculitis can cause numbness or weakness in your hands or feet, along with swollen or hardened palms and soles.

Lungs: If vasculitis affects your lungs, you could have shortness of breath or maybe cough up blood.

Genitals: Vasculitis in this area can cause ulcers or open sores.

Nose: Along with sinus infections and a runny nose, you could also get blisters in your nose.

Mouth: Vasculitis can make your lips and tongue swollen and dry, or your mouth and throat swell.

Diagnosis

Your doctor likely will start by taking your medical history and performing a physical exam. He or she may have you undergo one or more diagnostic tests and procedures to either rule out other conditions that mimic vasculitis or diagnose vasculitis. Tests and procedures might include:

Blood tests: These tests look for signs of inflammation, such as a high level of C-reactive protein. A complete blood cell count can tell whether you have enough red blood cells. Blood tests that look for certain antibodies — such as the anti-neutrophil cytoplasmic antibody (ANCA) test — can help diagnose vasculitis.

Imaging tests: Noninvasive imaging techniques can help determine which blood vessels and organs are affected. They can also help the doctor monitor whether you are responding to treatment. Imaging tests for vasculitis include X-rays, ultrasound, computerized tomography (CT), magnetic resonance imaging (MRI) and positron emission tomography (PET).

X-rays of your blood vessels (angiography): During this procedure, a flexible catheter, resembling a thin straw, is inserted into a large artery or vein. A special dye is then injected into the catheter, and X-rays are taken as the dye fills the artery or vein. The outlines of your blood vessels are visible on the resulting X-rays.

Biopsy: This is a surgical procedure in which your doctor removes a small sample of tissue from the affected area of your body. Your doctor then examines this tissue for signs of vasculitis.

Vasculitis Treatment

Which vasculitis treatment your doctor recommends depends on what's causing it and which organs it affects. It's usually meant to control the inflammation and prevent organ and blood vessel damage.

Medications

Steroids like prednisone are the most common medications prescribed to fight the inflammation vasculitis causes. Your doctor will watch you closely for side effects like high blood pressure, high blood sugar, and bone problems, especially if you take them for a long time.

Other medications, like azathioprine (Azasan, Imuran), cyclophosphamide (Cytoxan), methotrexate (Rheumatrex, Trexall), mycophenolate (CellCept, Myfortic), rituximab (Riabni, Rituxan, Ruxience, Truxima), or tocilizumab (Actemra) can be prescribed along with steroids. Which medication you might need depends on how serious your vasculitis is, whether it's in your organs, and your medical history.

Surgery

Sometimes vasculitis can cause issues that need surgery to repair. For instance, if your blood vessel walls bulge and form an aneurysm, surgery can lower the chances that it will burst. If you have a blocked artery, you could need surgery to restore blood flow to the area. But any kind of organ damage might require surgery.

Vasculitis Prognosis

There's no cure for vasculitis, but with the right treatment, you can live a long and active life. Most types of vasculitis are lifelong. But successful treatment can give you long periods without symptoms (called remissions).

Your outlook depends on several things, including:

- The type of vasculitis you have
- How quickly you were diagnosed
- Which organs are affected and how seriously
- Other health problems you have

2

IMPACT OF INFLAMMATION ON THE BODY

Inflammation is your body's response to an illness, injury or something that doesn't belong in your body (like germs or toxic chemicals). Inflammation is a normal and important process that allows your body to heal. Fever, for example, is how you know your body's inflammatory system is working correctly when you're ill. But inflammation can harm you if it occurs in healthy tissues or goes on for too long.

When an invader (like a virus) tries to enter your body, or you get injured, your immune system sends out its first responders. These are inflammatory cells and cytokines (substances that stimulate more inflammatory cells). These cells begin an inflammatory response to trap germs or toxins and start healing injured tissue. Inflammation can cause pain, swelling or discoloration. These are signs your body is healing itself. Normal inflammation should be mild, and pain shouldn't be extreme.

But inflammation can also affect parts of your body you can't see. Inflammatory responses that occur behind the scenes can help you heal, but other times, they can harm your health.

Types of Inflammation

There are two types of inflammation: acute and chronic.

Acute inflammation is the body's immediate response to an injury or infection. When the body is damaged, the immune system sends white blood cells to destroy any damaging substances, heal the tissues, and return the affected area to a state of balance. This rapid response causes familiar symptoms like redness, pain, warmth, and swelling. Acute inflammation usually resolves within a few hours to days.

Chronic inflammation can begin via the same process as acute inflammation but becomes persistent. It can happen in several ways. One possibility is that the threat remains because the body can't rid itself of the offending substance. Another scenario is that the immune system goes into "threat mode" when no actual threat exists. As a result, rather than healing tissues, the body breaks them down. Unhealthful lifestyle choices, such as smoking, a poor diet, excessive alcohol consumption, sedentary behavior, stress, and weight gain also can contribute to chronic inflammation.

Is inflammation helpful or harmful?

It turns out inflammation is both good and bad. On the one hand, acute inflammation helps the body to repair tissue damage and fight infections. Yet there is another side of inflammation that can be harmful rather than helpful to human health. A growing body of evidence suggests that low-grade, chronic inflammation contributes to some of the nation's leading killers, including cardiovascular disease, cancer, and type 2 diabetes as well as Alzheimer's disease, allergies and asthma, arthritis, anxiety and depression, and some skin conditions.

Where does inflammation occur?

Chronic inflammation can attack the entire body and, in the process, raise the risk for certain types of diseases and disorders in specific areas like the heart, brain, joints, and gastrointestinal tract.

Heart: Inflammation can raise the risk of heart attacks, and the link is believed to be related to cholesterol. Cholesterol can cause plaque build-up in the arteries, potentially blocking blood flow and leading to a heart attack. As cholesterol invades the wall of an artery, the immune system treats it like any other invader and releases inflammation-producing chemicals to help remove it. A fibrous cap is formed over the plaque. Inflammation inside the plaque can eventually eat away at the cap, and if it ruptures, the cholesterol, inflammatory cells, and chemicals in the plaque spill into the artery causing a blood clot to form which blocks blood flow.

Brain: Research has found that high amounts of inflammation in the body are associated with brain aging, increased cognitive decline, and "brain fog," which can impair thinking and cause memory lapses and confusion. Inflammation also may play a role in the production of an abnormal protein called tau, which is associated with Alzheimer's disease.

Joints: Chronic inflammation can lead to pain, swelling, stiffness, and joint damage, known as inflammatory arthritis. This can damage cartilage, bones, tendons (which attach muscle to bones), or ligaments (which hold joints together) and irritate nerves. Common types of inflammatory arthritis include rheumatoid arthritis, gout, and psoriatic arthritis.

Gastrointestinal tract: Inflammation is a driver of inflammatory bowel disease (IBD), a chronic inflammation of the gastrointestinal (GI) tract, including the stomach, gallbladder, and small and large intestines. Two types of IBD are ulcerative colitis, marked by continuous inflammation of the large intestine, and Crohn's disease, which causes inflammation anywhere in the GI tract. People with IBD can experience various symptoms, such as abdominal pain, diarrhea, blood in their stool, bloating, and weight loss.

Liver inflammation: Nonalcoholic fatty liver disease is fatty liver not caused by alcohol intake. There are two types: simple fatty liver and nonalcoholic steatohepatitis (NASH). Simple fatty liver doesn't cause inflammation. However, NASH is more severe and occurs when fattened cells become inflamed. This inflammation can damage liver cells, resulting in cirrhosis (permanent scarring of the liver), and increase the risk of liver cancer. Chronic liver inflammation can also be caused by a hepatitis C infection and lead to cirrhosis.

How do you reduce inflammation?

Although inflammation is vital to the body's defense and repair systems, chronic inflammation can cause more harm than good. That may make you wonder: what can I do about it? There are actually several ways to treat and reduce chronic inflammation. For example:

Follow a healthy, anti-inflammatory diet. Eating foods that have an anti-inflammatory effect may reduce inflammation and lower the risk of chronic illnesses associated with inflammation. Foods that reduce inflammation include:

tomatoes

olive oil

green leafy vegetables, such as spinach, kale, and collards

nuts like almonds and walnuts

fatty fish like salmon, mackerel, tuna, and sardines

whole grains such as quinoa, whole-grain bread, and oatmeal

fruits such as strawberries, blueberries, and oranges

These foods contain high amounts of anti-inflammatory compounds and antioxidants like carotenoids, polyphenols, and omega-3 fatty acids.

An easy way to eat more anti-inflammatory foods is to follow an eating plan like the Mediterranean and MIND diets, which emphasize these foods. Following an anti-inflammatory diet also helps you avoid unhealthy foods that can cause inflammation, such as refined carbohydrates, such as white bread and pastries, processed foods, sugar-sweetened beverages, and red meat. High amounts of these foods also contribute to weight gain, another risk factor for inflammation.

Other ways you can reduce inflammation include:

Regular exercise: Moderate-intensity exercise can help prevent excess weight gain and manage cytokine levels. Cytokines are small proteins that play an essential role in normal immune responses, but large amounts can lead to inflammation.

Manage stress: Repeated bouts of stress can expose the body to high levels of cortisol (the stress hormone) and lead to chronic inflammation. Yoga, deep breathing, meditation, and other forms of relaxation can help calm your nervous system.

Medications: Anti-inflammatory medicines can help treat inflammatory conditions. Examples include corticosteroids and over-the-counter nonsteroidal anti-inflammatory drugs, such as Ibuprofen and naproxen. Speak with your doctor about whether medication is an option because they could cause side effects.

3

THE ROLE OF DIET IN VASCULITIS MANAGEMENT

An anti-inflammatory diet is designed to reduce chronic inflammation, a key factor in various health conditions such as vasculitis. By focusing on specific nutrients and foods, this diet can play a crucial role in managing and alleviating inflammation-related symptoms.

Dietary Principles

To manage inflammation, it is essential to adopt dietary principles that support overall health.

A diet centered on whole, minimally processed foods is ideal.

This includes an ample variety of fruits and vegetables, which provide antioxidants and phytochemicals that help mitigate inflammation.

Whole grains are also a cornerstone of an anti-inflammatory diet as they are high in fiber, which aids in digestion and can help reduce inflammatory markers.

Consumption of proteins should be from lean sources, including fish rich in omega-3 fatty acids, like salmon and mackerel, which are known for their anti-inflammatory properties.

In addition to fish, other healthy protein sources such as legumes (beans, lentils) and nuts and seeds are encouraged.

Olive oil, a monounsaturated fat, is recommended as the primary fat source due to its potential to reduce inflammation.

Incorporating spices like turmeric, known for its curcumin content, can further assist in reducing inflammation.

This diet minimizes the intake of processed foods, sugary beverages, and refined carbohydrates, as these can exacerbate inflammation.

Key Nutrients and Foods

When adhering to an anti-inflammatory diet, focus on the following key nutrients and foods:

Omega-3 fatty acids: Found in fatty fish such as salmon and sardines, as well as in flaxseeds and walnuts, these fatty acids are vital for combating inflammation.

Antioxidants: A variety of colorful fruits and vegetables like berries, broccoli, and squash provide antioxidants that protect against cellular damage.

Fiber: High-fiber foods including whole grains, fruits and vegetables, and legumes help to reduce inflammation and support a healthy gut.

Healthy fats: Utilizing olive oil for cooking and dressings can provide the healthy fats critical for managing inflammation.

Herbs and spices: Using spices like turmeric in cooking can offer anti-inflammatory benefits due to compounds like curcumin.

Specific Dietary Recommendations

In managing vasculitis through diet, one focuses on anti-inflammatory foods that support overall health and reduce the body's inflammatory response.

It's important to discern what to include and avoid in your diet for optimal management of this condition.

Patients with high blood pressure should limit their intake of saturated fat, sodium, red meat, sweets, and beverages containing sugar. Instead, their diet should include:

Fruits

Vegetables

Whole grains

Low-fat dairy products

Skinless poultry and fish

Nuts and legumes

Non-tropical vegetable oils

Foods to Include and Avoid

Foods to Include

Mediterranean Diet: This diet emphasizes consuming fruits, vegetables, whole grains, legumes, nuts, and seeds.

It is also rich in mono- and polyunsaturated fats, such as those found in olive oil, which are known to have anti-inflammatory properties. Here are the components that should be included liberally:

Omega-3 Fatty Acids: Found in fatty fish, flaxseeds, and walnuts, omega-3s help reduce inflammation.

Antioxidants: Fruits and vegetables, like berries and leafy greens, are packed with antioxidants which combat inflammation.

Recommended Foods:

Fruits and Vegetables: Focus on a variety, including leafy greens and berries for their anti-inflammatory benefits.

Whole Grains: Opt for grains like quinoa, brown rice, and oats, which are less likely to promote inflammation.

Healthy Fats: Include sources of healthy fats such as avocados, olive oil, and nuts.

Foods to Avoid

Processed Foods and Saturated Fats: These foods can exacerbate inflammation and should be limited in an anti-inflammatory diet. This includes:

Processed Food: Anything heavily processed or with added preservatives should be avoided.

Saturated Fat: Foods high in saturated fat like butter and fatty cuts of meat can increase inflammation.

Salt: Excessive salt intake can worsen inflammation and strain on blood vessels.

Refined Sugars and Simple Carbohydrates: Consumption of these can lead to spikes in blood sugar and insulin levels, which may trigger an inflammatory response.

Specific Avoidances:

Sugar: Minimize intake of sugars that can prompt an inflammatory process.

Cookies and Sweets: These often contain both refined sugars and saturated fats, which are best avoided in an anti-inflammatory diet.

Managing Sodium Intake

Patients who have AAV with kidney disease benefit from a diet with limited sodium. Their sodium intake should be less than 2300 mg/d. Some tips for reducing sodium intake include:

Avoiding processed foods, which often contain high levels of sodium

Using herbs and spices rather than salt to add flavor to foods

Choosing low-sodium versions of foods such as canned vegetables and soups

Consuming the right amounts and types of protein

Limiting the consumption of saturated and trans fats

Patients with diabetes should eat a variety of healthful foods, including vegetables, fruits, grains, protein, and dairy. The amount of each should be specified in a meal plan. Foods to limit include those high in saturated and trans fats, sodium, and sugar.

Medical Treatments and Diet Interaction

When managing vasculitis, it's crucial to understand how medical treatments interact with dietary choices. Given the complexity of the medications often prescribed, dietary considerations play a significant role in optimizing treatment efficacy and minimizing side effects.

Medication Adjustments

Specific medications used in the treatment of vasculitis, such as corticosteroids (e.g., prednisone) and immunosuppressive agents like azathioprine, cyclophosphamide, and methotrexate, require careful monitoring by healthcare professionals.

Adjustments to these medications may become necessary based on a patient's response to treatment and any dietary changes they undertake.

For instance, corticosteroids can elevate blood sugar levels, necessitating adjustments in both the medication and dietary intake for those at risk of diabetes.

• Steroid use often requires:

• Increased calcium intake due to the risk of bone density loss.

• Monitoring of blood sugar levels due to increased risk of hyperglycemia.

• Cyclophosphamide treatment may involve:

• Hydration strategies to prevent bladder complications.

• Dietary changes to alleviate gastrointestinal side effects.

Dietary Considerations during Treatment

While undergoing treatment for vasculitis, dietary considerations can have a profound impact on the patient's well-being.

The inflammation associated with vasculitis may be exacerbated by certain foods; consequently, a diet low in processed foods and refined sugars is recommended.

Incorporating anti-inflammatory foods like leafy greens and omega-3 rich fish can support the body's ability to modulate inflammation.

Furthermore, patients receiving methotrexate are advised to increase their intake of folate-rich foods due to the medication's tendency to deplete folate stores in the body.

Lastly, those preparing for or recovering from surgery may require a tailored diet to ensure proper healing and to mitigate any potential side effects of the treatment.

4

VASCULITIS DIET RECIPES YOU MUST TRY!

DELIGHTFUL RECIPES FOR BREAKFAST

Orange & blueberry Bircher

Ingredients

• 70g porridge oats

• 2 tbsp golden linseeds

• zest of ½ an orange

• ¾ of a 175g tub yogurt

• 2 peeled and chopped oranges

• 4handfuls blueberries from a 150g pack

Directions

• STEP 1

Mix 70g oats and 2 tbsp golden linseeds with the zest of 1 /2 an orange. Pour over 300ml boiling water and leave overnight. The next day, stir in three-quarters of a 175g tub of yogurt, spoon into glasses or bowls, top with 2 peeled and chopped oranges, the remaining yogurt and 4 handfuls blueberries from a 150g pack.

Spicy Moroccan eggs

Ingredients

• 2 tsp rapeseed oil

• 1 large onion, halved and thinly sliced

• 3 garlic cloves, sliced

- 1 tbsp rose harissa

- 1 tsp ground coriander

- 150ml vegetable stock

- 400g can chickpea

- 2 x 400g cans cherry tomatoes

- 2 courgettes, finely diced

- 200g bag baby spinach

- 4 tbsp chopped coriander

- 4 large eggs

Directions

- STEP 1

Heat the oil in a large, deep frying pan, and fry the onion and garlic for about 8 mins, stirring every now and then, until starting to turn golden. Add the harissa and ground coriander, stir well, then pour in the stock and chickpeas with their liquid. Cover and simmer for 5 mins, then mash about one-third of the chickpeas to thicken the stock a little.

• STEP 2

Tip the tomatoes and courgettes into the pan, and cook gently for 10 mins until the courgettes are tender. Fold in the spinach so that it wilts into the pan.

• STEP 3

Stir in the chopped coriander, then make 4 hollows in the mixture and break in the eggs. Cover and cook for 2 mins, then take off the heat and allow to settle for 2 mins before serving.

Fig, nut & seed bread with ricotta & fruit

Ingredients

• 400ml hot strong black tea

• 100g dried fig, hard stalks removed, thinly sliced

• 140g sultana

• 50g porridge oat

• 200g self-raising wholemeal flour

• 1 tsp baking powder

• 100g mixed nuts (almonds, walnuts, Brazils, hazelnuts), plus 50g for the topping

• 1 tbsp golden linseed

• 1 tbsp sesame seed, plus 2 tsp to sprinkle

• 25g pumpkin seed

• 1 large egg

• 25g ricotta per person

• 1 orange or green apple, thickly sliced, per person

Directions

• STEP 1

Heat oven to 170C/150C fan/gas 3½. Pour the tea into a large bowl and stir in the figs, sultanas and oats. Set aside to soak.

• STEP 2

Meanwhile, line the base and sides of a 1kg loaf tin with baking parchment. Mix together the flour, baking powder, nuts and seeds. Beat the egg into the cooled fruit mixture, then stir the dry

Ingredients into the wet. Pour into the tin, then level the top and scatter with the extra nuts and sesame seeds.

• STEP 3

Bake for 1 hr, then cover the top with foil and bake for 15 mins more until a skewer inserted into the centre of the loaf comes out clean. Remove from the tin to cool, but leave the parchment on until cold. Cut into slices, spread with ricotta and serve with fruit. Will keep in the fridge for 1 month, or freeze in slices.

Staffordshire oatcakes with mushrooms

Ingredients

For the oatcakes

• 85g porridge oats

• 85g plain wholemeal flour

• ½ tsp dried yeast

For the topping

• 4 tsp rapeseed oil, plus a little for frying

• 320g button mushrooms, sliced

• 4 tomatoes, each cut into 8 wedges

• 4 tbsp milled seeds with flax and chia

• 4 tbsp tahini

• A few coriander sprigs, chopped

Directions

• STEP 1

For the oatcakes, tip the oats and 350ml water into
a bowl and blitz with a stick blender until smooth

(alternatively you can use a food processor or liquidizer). Stir in the flour and yeast, cover and leave in the fridge overnight, or leave at room temperature for 2-3 hrs until bubbles appear.

• STEP 2

Use kitchen paper to rub ½ tsp oil round a non-stick frying pan, then heat. Ladle in a quarter of the batter and swirl the pan to cover the base (the oatcakes should be a few millimeters thick, like a crêpe). Cook for 2 mins, then turn and cook for 2 mins more until golden. Make four oatcakes in the same way. If you're following our Healthy Diet Plan, chill two for another day. Will keep, covered in the fridge, for two days.

• STEP 3

To make the topping for two oatcakes, heat 2 tsp oil in a non-stick pan, add 160g mushrooms and fry for

2-3 mins, stirring until softened. Stir in 2 tomatoes, then add 2 tbsp ground seeds and cook for 2 mins more. Reheat the oatcakes in a dry frying pan or the microwave if necessary, then spread each one with 1 tbsp tahini, the mushroom mixture and scatter with a little coriander before serving. On the second day, repeat step 3 with the remaining Ingredients.

Orange & raspberry granola

Ingredients

• 400g jumbo oats

• juice 2 oranges (150ml), plus zest of 1/2

• 1 tsp ground cinnamon

• 2 tbsp freeze-dried raspberries or strawberries (see tip)

• 25g flaked almonds, toasted

• 25g mixed seeds (such as sunflower, pumpkin, sesame and linseed)

To serve

• 2 large oranges, peeled and segmented

• mint leaves (optional)

Directions

• STEP 1

Put 200g oats and 500ml water in a food processor and blitz for 1 min. Line a sieve with clean muslin and pour in the oat mixture. Leave to drip through for 5 mins, then twist the ends of the muslin and squeeze well to capture as much of the oat milk as possible – it should be the consistency of single cream. Best chilled at least 1 hr before serving. Can be kept in a sealed or covered jug in the fridge for up to 3 days.

• STEP 2

Heat oven to 200C/180C fan/gas 6 and line a baking tray with baking parchment. Put the orange juice in a medium saucepan and bring to the boil. Boil rapidly for 5 mins or until the liquid has reduced by half, stirring occasionally. Mix the remaining 200g oats with the orange zest and cinnamon. Remove the pan from the heat and stir the oat mixture into the juice. Spread over the lined tray in a thin layer and bake for 10-15 mins or until lightly browned and crisp, turning the oats every few mins. Leave to cool on the tray.

• STEP 3

Once cool, mix the oats with the raspberries, flaked almonds and seeds. Can be kept in a sealed jar for up to one week. To serve, spoon the granola into bowls, pour over the oat milk and top with the orange segments and mint leaves, if you like.

Green fritters

Ingredients

• 140g courgettes, grated

• 3 medium eggs

• 85g broccoli florets, finely chopped

• small pack dill, roughly chopped

• 3 tbsp gluten-free flour or rice flour

• 2 tbsp sunflower oil, for frying

Directions

• STEP 1

Squeeze the courgettes between your hands to remove any excess moisture, or tip onto a clean tea towel and twist it to squeeze out the moisture.

• STEP 2

Beat the eggs in a bowl, add the broccoli, courgettes and most of the dill, and mix together. Add the flour, mix again and season.

• STEP 3

Heat the oil in a non-stick frying pan. Put a large serving spoon of the mixture in the pan, then add 2 more spoonfuls so you have 3 fritters. Leave for 3-4 mins on a medium heat until golden brown on one side and solid enough for you to flip over, then flip over and leave to go golden on the other side.

Repeat to make 3 more fritters (there is no need to add any more oil to the pan after the first batch). Scatter with the remaining dill to serve.

Overnight oats with apricots & yogurt

Ingredients

For the oats

• 200g oats

• 50g chia seeds

• 1 tbsp vanilla extract

• 550ml almond milk, or cow's milk (if non-vegan)

For the apricots

• 1 tsp rapeseed oil

* 320g pack fresh apricots, stoned and quartered

* 400g pot fortified oat or plain bio yogurt

* 4 tsp sunflower seeds

Directions

* STEP 1

Mix the oats and chia in a bowl with the vanilla and almond milk. Cover and chill overnight.

* STEP 2

Heat the oil in a small non-stick pan. Add the apricots in a single layer, then cover the pan and cook over a low heat for 5 mins, until softened. Stir well and cook a few minutes more if needed – they will cook a little more in the residual heat as they cool. Cover and keep chilled until needed.

• STEP 3

The next day, stir the yogurt into the oats and spoon into tumblers, small jars or small bowls. Top with the cooked apricots and sunflower seeds. Will keep covered and chilled for up to four days.

Pancakes for one

Ingredients

• 1 large egg

• 40g plain flour

• ½ tsp baking powder

• 45ml milk (dairy, nut or oat based)

• 1 tsp butter

• ½ tbsp oil

• maple syrup or honey and berries, to serve (optional)

Directions

• STEP 1

Separate the egg, putting the white and yolk in separate bowls. Mix the egg yolk with the flour, baking powder and milk to make a smooth paste.

• STEP 2

Beat the egg white and a pinch of salt with an electric whisk (or by hand) until fluffy and holding its shape. Gently fold the egg white into the yolk mixture. Be extra careful not to knock any of the air out.

• STEP 3

Heat the butter and oil in a non-stick frying pan. Dollop a third of the mixture into the pan and cook on each side for 1-2 mins or until golden brown. Repeat with the remaining mixture to make three pancakes. Drizzle over some maple syrup or honey and serve with berries, if you like.

Dippy eggs with Marmite soldiers

Ingredients

• 2 eggs

• 4 slices wholemeal bread

• a knob of butter

• Marmite

• mixed seeds

Directions

• STEP 1

Bring a pan of water to a simmer. Add 2 eggs, simmer for 2 mins if room temp, 3 mins if fridge-cold, then turn off heat. Cover the pan and leave for 2 mins more.

• STEP 2

Meanwhile, toast 4 slices wholemeal bread and spread thinly with butter, then Marmite. To serve, cut into soldiers and dip into the egg, then a few mixed seeds.

Rye bread with almond butter & pink grapefruit segments

Ingredients

• 4 tbsp almond butter (make your own with the 'goes well with' recipe, right)

• 1 grapefruit (you will need about 100g flesh)

• 2 slices rye bread, toasted (optional)

Directions

• STEP 1

Toast your rye bread, if you like. Segment the grapefruit and spoon the fruit, along with any juice, into a small bowl.

• STEP 2

Spread the almond butter onto the rye bread, and top with the grapefruit, drizzling any juice over the top.

Creamy yogurt porridge with apricot, ginger & grapefruit topping

Ingredients

For the topping

• 300g can apricot in fruit juice

• 1 tsp finely grated ginger

• 2 pink grapefruits, segmented, any juice reserved

For the porridge

• 9 tbsp (75g) porridge oat

• 550g pot 0% fat probiotic plain yogurt

Directions

• STEP 1

For the topping: Tip the apricots and juice into a bowl, add ginger. Blitz half the mixture to a purée with a hand blender. Stir in the grapefruit and juice. Can be made ahead and chilled for up to 1 week.

• STEP 2

For the porridge: Tip 200ml water into a small non-stick pan and stir in porridge oats. Cook over a low heat until bubbling and thickened. (To make in a microwave, use a deep container to prevent spillage as the mixture will rise up as it cooks, and cook for 3 mins on High.) Stir in yogurt – or swirl in half and top with the rest. Top with the apricot mix.

Wholewheat flatbreads with beans & poached egg

Ingredients

• 2 eggs

For the beans

- 500g carton passata

- 2 small onions, quartered

- 1 medjool date, stoned

- 3 tsp smoked paprika

- 1 tsp balsamic vinegar

- 400g can haricot beans, drained

For the flatbreads .

- 100g wholewheat flour

- ½ tsp baking powder

- 100g natural yogurt

Directions

- STEP 1

Tip the passata into a food processor with the onions, date and paprika, and blitz until completely smooth. Heat in a medium pan, cover and simmer for 10 mins, stirring frequently, to make a thick pulpy sauce. Taste to make sure the onion is fully cooked. If not, add a splash of water and cook a little longer. Stir in the vinegar and beans, then remove from the heat.

• STEP 2

To make the flatbreads, tip the flour and baking powder into a bowl, then stir in the yogurt to make a soft dough. Tip out onto a lightly floured surface and lightly knead, fully incorporating any flour left in the bowl. Halve the mixture and flatten each piece to a rough oval, using your hands or a rolling pin, to a thickness of two £1 coins. Cut slashes through the centre of the ovals a couple of times with a sharp knife, being careful not to cut through an edge.

• STEP 3

Heat a large, non-stick pan, add a flatbread and cook for 1 min each side until firm and slightly puffed, then repeat with the other. Meanwhile, heat a large pan of water and poach the eggs to your liking.

• STEP 4

Warm the beans and serve on top of each flatbread with a poached egg and some black pepper.

Seven-cup muesli

Ingredients

• 3 cups oats

• 1 cup mixed nuts including macadamia if possible

• ½ cup sesame seeds

• ½ cup sunflower seeds

• ½ cup raisins

• ½ cup dried cranberries

• 1 cup dried ready-to-eat apricots, chopped

To serve

• soya or semi-skimmed milk

• chopped fresh seasonal fruit, such as pears, banana, pineapple, papya, passion fruit and grapes

Directions

• STEP 1

Tip the oats into a large airtight container and add the nuts, seeds, raisins and cranberries. Stir in the apricots.

• STEP 2

To serve, spoon a portion into a bowl, pour over the milk and top with chopped fresh fruit.

DELIGHTFUL RECIPES FOR LUNCH

Summer pistou

Ingredients

• 1 tbsp rapeseed oil

• 2 leeks, finely sliced

• 1 large courgette, finely diced

• 1l boiling vegetable stock (made from scratch or with reduced-salt bouillon)

• 400g can cannellini or haricot beans, drained

• 200g green beans, chopped

• 3 tomatoes, chopped

• 3 garlic cloves, finely chopped

• small pack basil

• 40g freshly grated parmesan

Directions

• STEP 1

Heat the oil in a large pan and fry the leeks and courgette for 5 mins to soften. Pour in the stock, add three-quarters of the haricot beans with the green beans, half the tomatoes, and simmer for 5-8 mins until the vegetables are tender.

• STEP 2

Meanwhile, blitz the remaining beans and tomatoes, the garlic and basil in a food processor (or in a bowl with a stick blender) until smooth, then stir in the Parmesan. Stir the sauce into the soup, cook for 1 min, then ladle half into bowls or pour into a flask for a packed lunch. Chill the remainder. Will keep for a couple of days.

Cod puttanesca with spinach & spaghetti

Ingredients

• 100g wholemeal spaghetti

• 1 large onion, sliced

• 1 tbsp rapeseed oil

• 1 red chilli, deseeded and sliced

• 2 garlic cloves, chopped

• 200g cherry tomatoes, halved

• 1 tsp cider vinegar

• 2 tsp capers

- 5 Kalamata olives, halved

- ½ tsp smoked paprika

- 2 skinless cod fillet or loins

- 160g spinach leaves

- small handful chopped parsley, to serve

Directions

- STEP 1

Boil the spaghetti for 10 mins until al dente, adding the spinach for the last 2 mins. Meanwhile, fry the onion in the oil in a large non-stick frying pan with a lid until tender and turning golden. Stir in the chilli and garlic, then add the tomatoes.

• STEP 2

Add the vinegar, capers, olives and paprika with a ladleful of the pasta water. Put the cod fillets on top, then cover the pan and cook for 5-7 mins until the fish just flakes. Drain the pasta and wilted spinach and pile on to plates, then top with the fish and sauce. Sprinkle over some parsley to serve.

Lentil Bolognese soup

Ingredients

• 2 tbsp rapeseed oil

• 3 onions, finely chopped

• 3 large carrots, finely diced

• 3 celery sticks, finely diced

* 4 garlic cloves, finely chopped

* 500g carton passata

* 1 tbsp vegetable bouillon powder

* 125g red lentils

* 1 tsp smoked paprika

* 4 sprigs fresh thyme

* 125g wholemeal penne

* 50g finely grated vegetarian Italian-style hard cheese

Directions

* STEP 1

Heat the oil in a large non-stick pan then fry the onions for a few mins until they start to colour. Add the carrots, celery and garlic then fry for 5 more mins, stirring frequently, until the vegetables start to soften.

• STEP 2

Pour in the passata, bouillon powder and the lentils with 2l boiling water. Add the smoked paprika, thyme and plenty of black pepper then bring to the boil, cover the pan and simmer for 20 mins.

• STEP 3

Tip in the penne then cook for 12-15 mins more until the pasta and lentils are tender, adding a little more water if necessary. Stir through the cheese, then ladle half the soup into bowls or a wide-necked flask if you're taking it as a packed lunch. Cool the remaining soup (remove the thyme sprigs) and keep in the fridge until required. It will keep well for several days. Reheat in a pan, adding a little extra water if the soup has thickened.

Summer egg salad with basil & peas

Ingredients

• 150g new potatoes, thickly sliced

• 160g French beans, trimmed

• 160g frozen peas

• 3 eggs

• 160g romaine lettuce, roughly torn into pieces

For the dressing

• 1 tbsp extra virgin olive oil

• 2 tsp cider vinegar

• ½ tsp English mustard powder

• 2 tbsp chopped mint

• 3 tbsp chopped basil

• 1 garlic clove, finely grated

• 1 tbsp capers

Directions

• STEP 1

Cook the potatoes in a pan of simmering water for 5 mins. Add the beans and cook 5 mins more, then tip in the peas and cook for 2 mins until all the vegetables are just tender. Meanwhile, boil the eggs in another pan for 8 mins. Drain and run under cold water, then carefully shell and halve.

• STEP 2

Mix all the dressing **Ingredients** together in a large bowl with a good grinding of black pepper, crushing the herbs and capers with the back of a spoon to intensify their flavours.

• STEP 3

Mix the warm vegetables into the dressing to coat, then add the lettuce and toss everything together. Pile onto plates, top with the eggs and grind over some black pepper to serve.

Butter bean curry wraps

Ingredients

• 2 large wholemeal tortilla wraps

• ½ the butter bean curry (recipe below)

• 2 handfuls of mixed salad leaves

• ½ the raita (recipe below)

Directions

• STEP 1

Warm the wraps following pack instructions, or for a few seconds on each side over the gas flame of the hob to create a slight char.

• STEP 2

Reheat leftover butter bean curry in a pan over a low heat until piping hot (if it's quite wet, allow it to reduce slightly). Spread the curry over the centre of the wraps, then top with the salad and the raita. Roll up tightly and serve straightaway.

Ingredients

- 1 lime, zested and juiced

- 1 small mango, stoned, peeled and chopped

- 1 small avocado, stoned, peeled and chopped

- 100g cherry tomatoes, halved

- 1 red chilli, deseeded and chopped

- 1 red onion, chopped

- ½ small pack coriander, chopped

- 400g can black beans, drained and rinsed

Directions

- STEP 1

Put the lime zest and juice, mango, avocado, tomatoes, chilli and onion in a bowl, stir through the coriander and beans.

Rustic vegetable soup

Ingredients

- 1 tbsp rapeseed oil

- 1 large onion, chopped

- 2 carrots, chopped

- 2 celery sticks, chopped

- 50g dried red lentils

- 1½ l boiling vegetable bouillon (we used Marigold)

- 2 tbsp tomato purée

- 1 tbsp chopped fresh thyme

- 1 leek, finely sliced

- 175g bite-sized cauliflower florets

• 1 courgette, chopped

• 3 garlic cloves, finely chopped

• ½ large Savoy cabbage, stalks removed and leaves chopped

• 1 tbsp basil, chopped

Directions

• STEP 1

Heat the oil in a large pan with a lid. Add the onion, carrots and celery and fry for 10 mins, stirring from time to time until they are starting to colour a little around the edges. Stir in the lentils and cook for 1 min more.

• STEP 2

Pour in the hot bouillon, add the tomato purée and thyme and stir well. Add the leek, cauliflower, courgette, and garlic, bring to the boil, then cover and leave to simmer for 15 mins.

• STEP 3

Add the cabbage and basil and cook for 5 mins more until the veg is just tender. Season with pepper, ladle into bowls and serve. Will keep in the fridge for a couple of days. Freezes well. Thaw, then reheat in a pan until piping hot.

Broccoli and kale green soup

Ingredients

• 500ml stock, made by mixing 1 tbsp bouillon powder and boiling water in a jug

• 1 tbsp sunflower oil

• 2 garlic cloves, sliced

• thumb-sized piece ginger, sliced

• ½ tsp ground coriander

• 3cm/1in piece fresh turmeric root, peeled and grated, or 1/2 tsp ground turmeric

• pinch of pink Himalayan salt

• 200g courgettes, roughly sliced

• 85g broccoli

• 100g kale, chopped

• 1 lime, zested and juiced

• small pack parsley, roughly chopped, reserving a few whole leaves to serve

Directions

• STEP 1

Put the oil in a deep pan, add the garlic, ginger, coriander, turmeric and salt, fry on a medium heat for 2 mins, then add 3 tbsp water to give a bit more moisture to the spices.

• STEP 2

Add the courgettes, making sure you mix well to coat the slices in all the spices, and continue cooking for 3 mins. Add 400ml stock and leave to simmer for 3 mins.

• STEP 3

Add the broccoli, kale and lime juice with the rest of the stock. Leave to cook again for another 3-4 mins until all the vegetables are soft.

• STEP 4

Take off the heat and add the chopped parsley. Pour everything into a blender and blend on high speed until smooth. It will be a beautiful green with bits of dark speckled through (which is the kale). Garnish with lime zest and parsley.

Spicy fish stew

Ingredients

- 1 tbsp olive oil

- 2 onions, thinly sliced

- 3 spring onions, chopped

- 3 garlic cloves, chopped

- 1 red chilli, seeded and thinly sliced

• few thyme sprigs

• 2 x 400g cans chopped tomatoes

• 400ml vegetable bouillon made with 2 tsp vegetable bouillon powder

• 2 green peppers, seeded and cut into pieces

• 160g brown basmati rice

• 400g can and 210g can red kidney beans, drained

• handful fresh coriander, chopped, plus a few sprigs extra

• handful flat-leaf parsley, chopped

• 550g pack frozen wild salmon, skinned and cut into large pieces

• 1 lime, zested

Directions

• STEP 1

Heat the oil in a large non-stick pan and fry the onions for 8-10 mins until softened and golden. Add the spring onions, garlic, chilli and thyme. Cook, stirring, for 1 min. Pour in the tomatoes and bouillon, then stir in the peppers. Cover and leave to simmer for 15 mins.

• STEP 2

Meanwhile, cook the rice according to pack instructions. Stir in the beans with the coriander and parsley, then leave to cook gently for another 10 mins until the peppers are tender. Add the salmon and lime zest and cook for 4-5 mins until cooked through.

• STEP 3

Ladle into bowls and scatter with the coriander sprigs.

Salmon salad with sesame dressing

Ingredients

For the salad

• 250g new potatoes, sliced

• 160g French beans, trimmed

• 2 wild salmon fillets

• 80g salad leaves

• 4 small clementines, 3 sliced, 1 juiced

• handful of basil, chopped

• handful of coriander, chopped

For the dressing

• 2 tsp sesame oil

• 2 tsp tamari

• ½ lemon, juiced

• 1 red chilli, deseeded and chopped

• 2 tbsp finely chopped onion (¼ small onion)

Directions

• STEP 1

Steam the potatoes and beans in a steamer basket set over a pan of boiling water for 8 mins. Arrange the salmon fillets on top and steam for a further 6-

8 mins, or until the salmon flakes easily when tested with a fork.

• STEP 2

Meanwhile, mix the dressing Ingredients together along with the clementine juice. If eating straightaway, divide the salad leaves between two plates and top with the warm potatoes and beans and the clementine slices. Arrange the salmon fillets on top, scatter over the herbs and spoon over the dressing. If taking to work, prepare the potatoes, beans and salmon the night before, then pack into a rigid airtight container with the salad leaves kept separate. Put the salad elements together and dress just before eating to prevent the leaves from wilting

Spaghetti puttanesca with red beans & spinach

Ingredients

• 100g wholemeal spaghetti

• 1 large onion, finely chopped

• 1 tbsp rapeseed oil

• 1 red chilli, deseeded and sliced

• 2 garlic cloves, chopped

• 200g cherry tomatoes, halved

• 2 tsp cider vinegar

• 1 tbsp capers

• 5 Kalamata olives, halved

• 1 tsp smoked paprika

• 210g can kidney beans, drained

• 160g spinach leaves

• small handful of chopped parsley

• small handful of basil leaves

Directions

• STEP 1

Cook the spaghetti in simmering water for 10-12 mins until al dente. Meanwhile, fry the onion in the oil in a large non-stick frying pan with a lid until tender and turning golden. Stir in the chilli, garlic and cherry tomatoes.

• STEP 2

Add the vinegar, capers, olives and paprika with a ladleful of pasta water. Stir in the beans and cook until warmed through.

• STEP 3

Add the spinach to the pasta water to wilt, then drain well. Toss with the tomato and bean mixture and the parsley and basil, then pile onto plates or in shallow bowls to serve.

Avocado & black bean eggs

Ingredients

• 2 tsp rapeseed oil

• 1 red chilli, deseeded and thinly sliced

• 1 large garlic clove, sliced

• 2 large eggs

• 400g can black beans

• ½ x 400g can cherry tomatoes

* ¼ tsp cumin seeds

* 1 small avocado, halved and sliced

* handful fresh, chopped coriander

* 1 lime, cut into wedges

Directions

* STEP 1

Heat the oil in a large non-stick frying pan. Add the chilli and garlic and cook until softened and starting to colour. Break in the eggs on either side of the pan. Once they start to set, spoon the beans (with their juice) and the tomatoes around the pan and sprinkle over the cumin seeds. You're aiming to warm the beans and tomatoes rather than cook them.

• STEP 2

Remove the pan from the heat and scatter over the avocado and coriander. Squeeze over half of the lime wedges. Serve with the remaining wedges on the side for squeezing over.

Spinach kedgeree with spiced salmon

Ingredients

• 2 tsp rapeseed oil

• 1 large onion, halved and sliced

• thumb-sized piece of ginger, finely chopped

• ½ tsp cumin seeds

• ½ tsp ground cinnamon

• 6-8 cardamom pods, seeds crushed

- 1½ tsp ground turmeric

- 1½ tsp ground coriander

- 1 red chilli, deseeded and sliced

- 1 garlic clove, finely chopped

- 1 large red pepper, deseeded and roughly chopped

- 70g brown basmati rice

- 375ml vegetable stock, made with 2 tsp bouillon powder

- 160g baby spinach leaves, roughly chopped

For the salmon

- 3 tbsp fat-free natural yogurt

- 1 tbsp finely chopped mint or coriander

- 2 skinless wild salmon fillets

• 1 tbsp toasted almonds, to serve

Directions

• STEP 1

Heat the oil in a large frying pan and fry the onion and ginger for 5 mins or until soft. Add the cumin, cinnamon, crushed cardamom seeds, and 1 tsp each of the turmeric and coriander. Cook for 30 secs until fragrant. Add the chilli, garlic, pepper and rice, stir briefly, then pour in the stock. Cover and simmer for 35 mins or until the rice is tender and the stock has been absorbed. If the rice is cooked but some liquid remains, remove the lid and simmer uncovered to allow the liquid to evaporate. Add the spinach, cover and cook for 3 mins to wilt.

• STEP 2

Meanwhile, prepare the salmon. Heat the grill to medium and line a baking sheet with foil. Mix the yogurt with the mint or coriander and the remaining turmeric and ground coriander. Spread the yogurt mixture over the salmon, then transfer to the prepared baking sheet and grill for 8-10 mins until the fish can be flaked easily with a fork. Top the kedgeree with the salmon fillets or flake the fish into it, and scatter over the almonds to serve.

DELIGHTFUL RECIPES FOR DINNER

Prawn & harissa spaghetti

Ingredients

• 100g long-stem broccoli, cut into thirds

• 180g dried spaghetti, regular or wholemeal

• 2 tbsp olive oil

• 1 large garlic clove, lightly bashed

• 150g cherry tomatoes, halved

• 150g raw king prawns

• 1 heaped tbsp rose harissa paste

• 1 lemon, finely zested

Directions

• STEP 1

Bring a pan of lightly salted water to the boil. Add the broccoli and boil for 1 min 30 secs, or until tender. Drain and set aside. Cook the spaghetti following pack instructions, then drain, reserving a ladleful of cooking water.

• STEP 2

Heat the oil in a large frying pan, add the garlic clove and fry over a low heat for 2 mins. Remove with a slotted spoon and discard, leaving the flavoured oil.

• STEP 3

Add the tomatoes to the pan and fry over a medium heat for 5 mins, or until beginning to soften and turn juicy. Stir through the prawns and cook for 2 mins, or until turning pink. Add the harissa and lemon zest, stirring to coat.

• STEP 4

Toss the cooked spaghetti and pasta water through the prawns and harissa. Stir through the broccoli, season to taste and serve.

Giant couscous salad with charred veg & tangy pesto

Ingredients

• 2-3 raw beetroot (320g), peeled and chopped

• 3 red onions (320g), cut into wedges

• 2 green or orange peppers, deseeded and cubed

• 1 tbsp olive oil

- 320g cherry tomatoes

- 200g wholewheat giant couscous

For the pesto

- 7g fresh coriander, roughly chopped

- 15g flat-leaf parsley, roughly chopped

- 1 garlic clove

- 1 green chilli, deseeded

- ½ tsp cumin

- 1 tbsp apple cider vinegar

- 1 tbsp olive oil

- 40g pine nuts, lightly toasted

Directions

• STEP 1

Heat the oven to 200C/180C fan/gas 6. In a bowl, toss the beetroot, onions and peppers together with the oil, then spread out on a large roasting tray lined with baking paper and roast for 35 mins. Scatter over the cherry tomatoes, then return to the oven for 10 mins more until the tomatoes have softened and the vegetables are tender.

• STEP 2

Meanwhile, cook the couscous following pack instructions, then rinse and drain. To make the pesto, put the coriander and half the parsley in a bowl with the garlic, chilli, cumin, vinegar, oil and 25g of the pine nuts. Add 2 tbsp water, then blitz with a hand blender until smooth or use a small food processor.

• STEP 3

Toss the roasted veg and chopped parsley through the couscous and pile on the pesto, then scatter with the remaining pine nuts.

Tomato penne with avocado

Ingredients

• 100g wholemeal penne

• 1 tsp rapeseed oil

• 1 large onion, sliced, plus 1 tbsp finely chopped

• 1 orange pepper, deseeded and cut into chunks

• 2 garlic cloves, grated

- 2 tsp mild chilli powder

- 1 tsp ground coriander

- ½ tsp cumin seeds

- 400g can chopped tomatoes

- 196g can sweetcorn in water

- 1 tsp vegetable bouillon powder

- 1 avocado, stoned and chopped

- 1/2 lime, zest and juice

- handful coriander, chopped, plus extra to serve

Directions

- STEP 1

Cook the pasta in salted water for 10-12 mins until al dente. Meanwhile, heat the oil in a medium pan.

Add the sliced onion and pepper and fry, stirring frequently for 10 mins until golden. Stir in the garlic and spices, then tip in the tomatoes, half a can of water, the corn and bouillon. Cover and simmer for 15 mins.

• STEP 2

Meanwhile, toss the avocado with the lime juice and zest, and the finely chopped onion.

• STEP 3

Drain the penne and toss into the sauce with the coriander. Spoon the pasta into bowls, top with the avocado and scatter over the coriander leaves.

Vegan carbonara

Ingredients

• 360g wholewheat spaghetti

• 85g unsalted cashew nuts

• 2 tsp bouillon powder

• 2 tsp English mustard powder

• 1 tsp olive oil

• 200g baby chestnut mushrooms, halved and thinly sliced

• 3 garlic cloves, 2 finely grated

• 1 tsp smoked paprika

• 2 courgettes (about 320g), peeled then grated

• 4 tsp nutritional yeast flakes, optional

• 320g spinach, half cooked each evening as a side dish

Directions

• STEP 1

Boil the spaghetti for 10 mins or following pack instructions until al dente, reserving a little of the water. Put the cashews, bouillon and mustard in a bowl, then pour over 350ml boiling water.

• STEP 2

Heat the oil in a large non-stick pan. Add the mushrooms and grated garlic, and stir-fry over a high heat until the mushrooms are cooked and starting to crisp up. Take off the heat, stir in the paprika, then tip onto a plate and set aside.

• STEP 3

Add the grated courgette to the pan and cook, stirring every now and then until softened. Meanwhile, whizz the soaked cashews, whole garlic clove and nutritional yeast flakes, if using, with a hand blender until completely smooth. Tip the mixture into the pan with the courgettes and briefly stir over the heat.

• STEP 4

Add the spaghetti and toss in the cashew and courgette mixture until well coated, then toss through the smoky mushrooms. erve half with half the spinach on the side, and chill the rest for another day. Will keep for three days. Reheat in a covered pan with a dash of water, and cook the remaining spinach to serve on the side.

Noodle salad with sesame dressing

Ingredients

For the dressing

• 1 tbsp sesame oil

• 2 tsp tamari

• 1 lemon, juiced

• 1 red chilli, deseeded and finely chopped

For the salad

• 1 small onion, finely chopped

• 2 wholemeal noodle nests (about 100g)

• 160g sugar snap peas

• 4 small clementines, peeled and chopped

• 160g shredded carrots

• large handful of coriander, chopped

• 50g roasted unsalted cashews

Directions

• STEP 1

Mix all the dressing Ingredients together in a large bowl, then stir in the onion. Meanwhile, cook the noodles in a pan of boiling water for 5 mins, adding the sugar snap peas halfway through the cooking time – the noodles and peas should be just tender. Drain, cool under cold running water and drain again. Snip or cut the noodles into smaller lengths to make them more manageable to eat.

• STEP 2

Tip the noodles and peas into the bowl with the dressing, along with the clementines, carrots, coriander and cashews. Toss to combine, then serve in bowls or pack into rigid airtight containers to take to work.

Minty griddled chicken & peach salad

Ingredients

• 1 lime, zested and juiced

• 1 tbsp rapeseed oil

• 2 tbsp mint, finely chopped, plus a few leaves to serve

• 1 garlic clove, finely grated

• 2 skinless chicken breast fillets (300g)

• 160g fine beans, trimmed and halved

• 2 peaches (200g), each cut into 8 thick wedges

• 1 red onion, cut into wedges

• 1 large Little Gem lettuce (165g), roughly shredded

• ½ x 60g pack rocket

• 1 small avocado, stoned and sliced

• 240g cooked new potatoes

Directions

• STEP 1

Mix the lime zest and juice, oil and mint, then put half in a bowl with the garlic. Thickly slice the chicken at a slight angle, add to the garlic mixture and toss together with plenty of black pepper.

• STEP 2

Cook the beans in a pan of water for 3-4 mins until just tender. Meanwhile, griddle the chicken and onion for a few mins each side until cooked and tender. Transfer to a plate, then quickly griddle the peaches. If you don't have a griddle pan, use a non-stick frying pan with a drop of oil.

• STEP 3

Toss the warm beans and onion in the remaining mint mixture, and pile onto a platter or into individual shallow bowls with the lettuce and rocket. Top with the avocado, peaches and chicken and scatter over the mint. Serve with the potatoes while still warm.

Meatballs with fennel & balsamic beans & courgette noodles

Ingredients

• 400g lean beef steak mince

• 2 tsp dried oregano

- 1 large egg

- 8 garlic cloves, 1 finely grated, the other sliced

- 1-2 tbsp olive oil

- 1 fennel bulb, finely chopped, fronds reserved

- 2 carrots, finely chopped

- 500g carton passata

- 4 tbsp balsamic vinegar

- 600ml reduced-salt vegetable bouillon

For the courgette noodles

- 1 tsp rapeseed oil

- 1-2 large courgettes, cut into noodles with a julienne peeler or spiralizer

- 350g frozen soya beans, thawed

Directions

• STEP 1

Put the mince, oregano, egg and grated garlic in a bowl and grind in some black pepper. Mix together thoroughly and roll into 16 balls.

• STEP 2

Heat the oil in a large sauté pan over a medium-high heat, add the meatballs and fry, moving them around the pan so that they brown all over – be careful as they're quite delicate and you don't want them to break up. Once brown, remove them from the pan. Reduce the heat slightly and add the fennel, carrots and sliced garlic to the pan and fry, stirring until they soften, about 5 mins.

• STEP 3

Tip in the passata, balsamic vinegar and bouillon, stir well, then return the meatballs to the pan, cover and cook gently for 20-25 mins.

• STEP 4

Meanwhile, heat the 1 tsp of oil in a non-stick pan and stir-fry the courgette with the beans to heat through and soften. Serve with the meatballs and scatter with any fennel fronds.

Cumin-spiced halloumi with corn & tomato slaw

Ingredients

• 1 lime, zested and juiced

• 1 tsp rapeseed oil

• 1 tsp fresh thyme leaves

• ¼ tsp turmeric

• ¼ tsp cumin seeds

• 1 tbsp finely chopped coriander

• 1 garlic clove, finely grated

• 100g halloumi, thinly sliced

For the slaw

• 1 lime, zested and juiced

• 3 tbsp bio yogurt

• 3 tbsp finely chopped coriander

• 1 red chilli, deseeded and chopped

• 160g corn, cut from 2 fresh cobs

• 1 red pepper, deseeded and chopped

• 100g fine green beans, blanched, trimmed and halved

• 200g cherry tomatoes, halved

• 1 red onion, halved and finely sliced

• 320g white cabbage, finely sliced

Directions

• STEP 1

Mix the lime zest and juice with the oil, thyme, turmeric, cumin, coriander and garlic together in a bowl. Add the halloumi and carefully turn it until coated – take care as it breaks easily.

• STEP 2

To make the slaw, mix the lime juice and zest, yogurt, coriander and chilli together, then stir in the corn, red pepper, beans, tomatoes, onion and cabbage.

• STEP 3

Heat a large non-stick frying pan or griddle pan and fry the cheese in batches for 1 min each side. Serve the slaw on plates with the halloumi slices on top. If you're cooking for two people, serve half of the halloumi and slaw and chill the rest for lunch another day.

Chicken & chorizo ragu

Ingredients

• 120g cooking chorizo, chopped

• 1 red onion, chopped

• 2 garlic cloves, grated

• 1 tsp hot smoked paprika

• 80g sundried tomatoes, roughly chopped

• 600g skinless and boneless chicken thighs

• 400g can chopped tomatoes

• 100ml chicken stock

• 1 lemon, juiced

• jacket potatoes, chopped parsley and soured cream, to serve (optional)

Directions

• STEP 1

Fry the chorizo over a medium heat in a large saucepan or flameproof casserole dish for 5 mins or until it releases its oil and starts to char at the edges. Add the onion and fry for 5 mins more or until soft. Tip in the garlic and cook for 2 mins before stirring in the paprika and sundried tomatoes. Add the chicken thighs and fry for 2 mins each side until they are well coated in the spices and beginning to brown.

• STEP 2

Pour in the chopped tomatoes and stock, and turn the heat down. Cover and cook for 40 mins until the chicken is falling apart and the sauce is thick. Stir the lemon juice through. Serve by piling spoonfuls of the ragu into hot jacket potatoes with parsley sprinkled over and a dollop of soured cream, if you like.

Spinach kedgeree with spiced salmon

Ingredients

• 2 tsp rapeseed oil

• 1 large onion, halved and sliced

• thumb-sized piece of ginger, finely chopped

• ½ tsp cumin seeds

- ½ tsp ground cinnamon

- 6-8 cardamom pods, seeds crushed

- 1½ tsp ground turmeric

- 1½ tsp ground coriander

- 1 red chilli, deseeded and sliced

- 1 garlic clove, finely chopped

- 1 large red pepper, deseeded and roughly chopped

- 70g brown basmati rice

- 375ml vegetable stock, made with 2 tsp bouillon powder

- 160g baby spinach leaves, roughly chopped

For the salmon

- 3 tbsp fat-free natural yogurt

• 1 tbsp finely chopped mint or coriander

• 2 skinless wild salmon fillets

• 1 tbsp toasted almonds, to serve

Directions

• STEP 1

Heat the oil in a large frying pan and fry the onion and ginger for 5 mins or until soft. Add the cumin, cinnamon, crushed cardamom seeds, and 1 tsp each of the turmeric and coriander. Cook for 30 secs until fragrant. Add the chilli, garlic, pepper and rice, stir briefly, then pour in the stock. Cover and simmer for 35 mins or until the rice is tender and the stock has been absorbed. If the rice is cooked but some liquid remains, remove the lid and simmer uncovered to allow the liquid to evaporate. Add the spinach, cover and cook for 3 mins to wilt.

• STEP 2

Meanwhile, prepare the salmon. Heat the grill to medium and line a baking sheet with foil. Mix the yogurt with the mint or coriander and the remaining turmeric and ground coriander. Spread the yogurt mixture over the salmon, then transfer to the prepared baking sheet and grill for 8-10 mins until the fish can be flaked easily with a fork. Top the kedgeree with the salmon fillets or flake the fish into it, and scatter over the almonds to serve.

Stir-fried chicken with broccoli & brown rice

Ingredients

• 200g trimmed broccoli florets (about 6), halved

• 1 chicken breast (approx 180g), diced

• 15g ginger, cut into shreds

- 2 garlic cloves, cut into shreds

- 1 red onion, sliced

- 1 roasted red pepper, from a jar, cut into cubes

- 2 tsp olive oil

- 1 tsp mild chilli powder

- 1 tbsp reduced-salt soy sauce

- 1 tbsp honey

- 250g pack cooked brown rice

Directions

- STEP 1

Put the kettle on to boil and tip the broccoli into a medium pan ready to go on the heat. Pour the water over the broccoli then boil for 4 mins.

• STEP 2

Heat the olive oil in a non-stick wok and stir-fry the ginger, garlic and onion for 2 mins, add the mild chilli powder and stir briefly. Add the chicken and stir-fry for 2 mins more. Drain the broccoli and reserve the water. Tip the broccoli into the wok with the soy, honey, red pepper and 4 tbsp broccoli water then cook until heated through. Meanwhile, heat the rice following the pack instructions and serve with the stir-fry.

Steaks with goulash sauce & sweet potato fries

Ingredients

• 3 tsp rapeseed oil, plus extra for the steaks

• 250g sweet potatoes, peeled and cut into narrow chips

- 1 tbsp fresh thyme leaves

- 2 small onions, halved and sliced (190g)

- 1 green pepper, deseeded and diced

- 2 garlic cloves, sliced

- 1 tsp smoked paprika

- 85g cherry tomatoes, halved

- 1 tbsp tomato purée

- 1 tsp vegetable bouillon powder

- 2 x 125g fillet steaks, rubbed with a little rapeseed oil

- 200g bag baby spinach, wilted in a pan or the microwave

Directions

- STEP 1

Heat oven to 240C/220C fan/gas 7 and put a wire rack on top of a baking tray. Toss the sweet potatoes and thyme with 2 tsp oil in a bowl, then scatter them over the rack and set aside until ready to cook.

- STEP 2

Heat 1 tsp oil in a non-stick pan, add the onions, cover the pan and leave to cook for 5 mins. Take off the lid and stir – they should be a little charred now. Stir in the green pepper and garlic, cover the pan and cook for 5 mins more. Put the potatoes in the oven and bake for 15 mins.

• STEP 3

While the potatoes are cooking, stir the paprika into the onions and peppers, pour in 150ml water and stir in the cherry tomatoes, tomato purée and bouillon. Cover and simmer for 10 mins.

• STEP 4

Pan-fry the steak in a hot, non-stick pan for 2-3 mins each side depending on their thickness. Rest for 5 mins. Spoon the goulash sauce onto plates and top with the beef. Serve the chips and spinach alongside.

DELIGHTFUL RECIPES FOR SNACK

Weaning recipe: Fish pie bites

Ingredients

• 1 medium baking potato

• 1 small salmon fillet, about 120g

• 1 tbsp frozen sweetcorn and peas, defrosted

• 1 tsp fresh chives, snipped into little strands

• 25g mild cheddar, grated

• ½ small egg, beaten

• oil, for greasing

Directions

• STEP 1

Heat the oven to 200C/ 180 fan/ gas 6. Wrap the potato in foil, place on a baking tray and roast in the oven for 1 hour 15 mins. Wrap the fish in foil, put on the same tray and continue cooking for around 10-12 mins until opaque and cooked through.

• STEP 2

Once cooked, halve the potato and scoop out the filling. Flake the fish, removing any bones and discarding the skin.

• STEP 3

Grease a baking tray with a little oil. Mash the potato, then mix through the flaked fish, veg, chives, cheese and egg. Allow to cool a little, then take golf-ball sized dollops of mixture and form into little croquette shapes. Arrange on a foil-lined tray and chill in the fridge for 30 mins. If freezing, put the tray in the freezer instead. Once frozen, transfer to a freezer bag and take them out when needed. Thoroughly defrost in the fridge before cooking.

• STEP 4

To cook, heat the oven to 200C/ 180 fan/ gas 6. Arrange as many as you need on a baking tray and cook for around 15 mins or until golden and cooked through. The inside will be very hot so make sure it's sufficiently cooled before serving to your little one.

Chia & almond overnight oats

Ingredients

• 200g jumbo porridge oats

• 50g chia seeds

• 600ml unsweetened almond milk, plus 8 tbsp

• 2 tsp vanilla extract

• 125g punnet raspberries

• 100g almond yogurt

• 250g punnet blueberries

• 20g flaked almonds, toasted

Directions

• STEP 1

Tip the oats and seeds into a bowl and pour over the milk and vanilla extract. Leave for 5-10 mins for the oats to absorb some of the liquid.

• STEP 2

Reserve 16 raspberries, then add the remainder to the oats and crush them into the mixture. Spoon into four tumblers or sundae dishes, then top with the yogurt and both lots of berries. Cover and chill overnight or until needed. To serve, pour 2 tbsp almond milk over each and scatter with the almonds.

Instant frozen berry yogurt

Ingredients

• 250g frozen mixed berry

• 250g Greek yogurt

• 1tbsp honey or agave syrup

Directions

• STEP 1

Blend berries, yogurt and honey or agave syrup in a food processor for 20 seconds, until it comes together to a smooth ice-cream texture. Scoop into bowls and serve.

Chia & oat breakfast scones with yogurt and berries

Ingredients

• 2 tsp cold pressed rapeseed oil, plus a little for the ramekins

• 50ml milk

• 1 tbsp lemon juice

• 2 tsp vanilla extract

• 160g plain wholemeal spelt flour

* 2 tbsp chia seeds

* 25g oats

* 2 tsp baking powder

* 2 x 120g pots bio Greek yogurt

* 400g strawberries, hulled and sliced

Directions

* STEP 1

Heat oven to 200C/180C fan/gas 6 and line the base of 4 x 185ml ramekins with a disc of baking parchment and oil the sides with the rapeseed oil. Measure the milk in a jug and make up to 300ml with water. Stir in the lemon juice, vanilla and the 2 tsp oil. Mix the flour, seeds and oats then blitz in a food processor to make the mix as fine as you can. Stir in the baking powder.

• STEP 2

Pour in the liquid, then stir in with the blade of a knife until you have a very wet batter like dough. Spoon evenly into the ramekins then bake on a baking sheet for 20 mins until risen – they don't have to be golden but should feel firm. Cool for a few mins then run a knife round the inside of the ramekins to loosen the scones then carefully ease out. The scones can be eaten immediately or cooled and stored for later.

Polenta bruschetta with tapenade

Ingredients

• 700ml vegetable stock (Marigold Swiss vegetable bouillon is gluten and dairy-free)

• 140g instant polenta

* 2 tbsp chopped fresh basil

* 2 tbsp olive oil

* 9 tsp (about half a 190g jar) olive tapenade

* 9 SunBlush or semi-dried tomatoes, halved

* 100g mixed salad leaves

Directions

* STEP 1

Bring the stock to the boil in a saucepan, then reduce to a simmer. Stirring continuously, pour in the polenta in a steady steam and cook for 5 mins until thickened. Stir in the basil and season with black pepper and salt, if you like. Spread on an oiled shallow tin measuring 24 x 18cm. Leave to set for 1 hr.

• STEP 2

Cut the polenta into 9 rectangles, each 8 x 6cm, then cut in half diagonally to make triangle shapes. Heat a griddle until hot, brush each triangle with oil and grill for 4-5 mins each side, until crisp and golden.

• STEP 3

Top each triangle with ½ tsp tapenade and half a tomato. Serve warm on salad leaves.

Quinoa porridge

Ingredients

For the porridge (to serve 4)

• 175g quinoa

• ½ vanilla pod, split and seeds scraped out, or 0.5 tsp vanilla extract

• 15g creamed coconut

• 4 tbsp chia seeds

• 125g coconut yogurt

For the topping (to serve 2)

• 125g pot coconut yogurt

• 280g mixed summer berries, such as strawberries, raspberries and blueberries

• 2 tbsp flaked almonds (optional)

Directions

• STEP 1

Activate the quinoa by soaking overnight in cold water. The next day, drain and rinse the quinoa through a fine sieve (the grains are so small that they will wash through a coarse one).

• STEP 2

Tip the quinoa into a pan and add the vanilla, creamed coconut and 600ml water. Cover the pan and simmer for 20 mins. Stir in the chia with another 300ml water and cook gently for 3 mins more. Stir in the pot of coconut yogurt. Spoon half the porridge into a bowl for another day. Will keep for 2 days covered in the fridge. Serve the remaining porridge topped with another pot of yogurt, the berries and almonds, if you like.

• STEP 3

To have the porridge another day, tip into a pan and reheat gently, with milk or water. Top with fruit - for instance, orange slices and pomegranate seeds.

Tuna Niçoise protein pot

Ingredients

• 1 large egg

• 80g green beans

• 1 tomato, amber or red, quartered

• 120g can tuna in spring water

• 1½ -2 tbsp French dressing

Directions

• STEP 1

Boil the egg for 8-10 mins depending on if you want a soft or hard yolk, then at the same time steam the green beans for 6 mins above the pan until tender. Cool the egg and beans under running water then carefully shell and quarter the egg. Leave to cool.

• STEP 2

Tip the beans into a large packed lunch pot. Top with the tomato, tuna and quartered egg and spoon on the French dressing. Seal until ready to eat.

Homemade vegan bagels

Ingredients

• 7g sachet dried yeast

• 4 tbsp sugar

• 2 tsp salt

• 450g bread flour

• poppy, fennel and/or sesame seeds to sprinkle on top (optional)

Directions

• STEP 1

Tip the yeast and 1 tbsp sugar into a large bowl, and pour over 100ml warm water. Leave for 10 mins until the mixture becomes frothy.

• STEP 2

Pour 200ml warm water into the bowl, then stir in the salt and half the flour. Keep adding the remaining flour (you may not have to use it all) and mixing with your hands until you have a soft but not sticky dough. Then knead for 10 mins until the dough feels smooth and elastic. Shape into a ball and put in a clean, lightly oiled bowl. Cover loosely and leave in a warm place until doubled in size, about 1hr.

• STEP 3

Heat the oven to 220C/200C fan/gas 7. On a lightly floured surface, divide the dough into 10 pieces, each about 85g. Shape each piece into a flattish ball, then take a wooden spoon and use the handle to make a hole in the middle of each ball. Slip the spoon into the hole, then twirl the bagel around the spoon to make a hole about 3cm wide. Cover the bagel loosely while you shape the remaining dough.

• STEP 4

Meanwhile, bring a large pan of water to the boil and tip in the remaining sugar. Slip the bagels into the boiling water – no more than four at a time. Cook for 1-2 mins, turning over in the water until the bagels have puffed slightly and a skin has formed. Remove with a slotted spoon and drain away any excess water. Sprinkle over your choice of topping and place on a baking tray lined with parchment. Bake in the oven for 25 mins until browned and crisp – the bases should sound hollow when tapped. Leave to cool on a wire rack, then serve with your favourite filling.

Puff pastry pizzas

Ingredients

• 320g sheet ready-rolled light puff pastry

• 6 tbsp tomato purée

• 1 tbsp tomato ketchup

• 1 tsp dried oregano

• 75g mozzarella or cheddar

For the topping

• sweetcorn, olives, peppers, red onion, cherry tomatoes, spinach, basil

Directions

• STEP 1

Heat the oven to 200C/180C fan/gas 6, or if using an air-fryer, heat it to 180C for 4 mins. Unroll the pastry, cut into six squares and arrange over two baking trays lined with baking parchment. Use a cutlery knife to score a 1cm border around the edge of each pastry square. Bake in the oven for 15 mins, until puffed up but not cooked through. Or, if using an air-fryer, bake the batch for 8 mins. You might need to do this in two batches.

• STEP 2

While the pastry cooks, make the sauce and prepare your toppings. Mix the tomato purée, tomato ketchup, oregano and 1 tbsp water. Grate the cheese and chop any veg or herbs you want to put on top into small pieces. Set aside.

• STEP 3

Remove the pastry from the oven or air-fryer and squash down the middles with the back of a spoon. Divide the sauce between the pastry squares and spread it out to the puffed-up edges. Sprinkle with the cheese, then add your toppings. Bake for another 5-8 mins in the oven or 5 mins in the air-fryer and serve.

Sweetcorn fritters

Ingredients

• 150g self-raising flour

• 1 tsp baking powder

* 1 tsp smoked paprika

* 160ml whole milk

* 1 egg

* 550g sweetcorn

* 2 spring onions, chopped, plus a little extra cut into thin strips to serve (optional)

* 10g sliced chives

* handful of parsley, chopped

* rapeseed oil, for frying

Directions

* STEP 1

Mix the flour, baking powder, paprika and milk together in a large bowl. Mix in the egg, followed by the sweetcorn, chopped spring onions, chives, parsley, 1 tsp salt and some freshly ground black pepper.

• STEP 2

Heat a 1cm depth of oil in a frying pan over a medium heat until a small amount of the fritter mixture sizzles when dropped in. For larger fritters, drop 2 heaped tablespoons of the mixture into the pan at a time in a clockwise direction (this will help you remember the order they were added to the pan, so you can flip them at the right stage). For smaller fritters, do the same, but with 1 heaped tablespoon of mixture at a time.

• STEP 3

After 2 mins, flip the fritters over in the same order they were added to the pan. Cook for another 2 mins, continuing to turn every now and then to ensure both sides are evenly golden brown. When ready, the fritters should be darker brown with crispy pieces of corn at the edges – be careful, as some of the kernels may burst during the cooking process. Remove to a wire rack and pat away any excess oil using kitchen paper. Serve straightaway with a few strips of spring onion scattered over, if you like.

Cheese-stuffed garlic dough balls with a tomato sauce dip

Ingredients

• 50g butter, cubed

• 300g strong white bread flour

• 7g sachet fast-action dried yeast

• 1 tbsp caster sugar

• 200g block mozzarella, cut into 1.5cm cubes

• 65g gruyère, coarsely grated (optional)

For the garlic butter

• 100g butter

• 2 garlic cloves, crushed

• 1 rosemary sprig, leaves picked and finely chopped

For the tomato sauce dip

• 1 tbsp olive oil, plus extra for the bowl and baking sheet

• 1 garlic clove, sliced

• 250g passata

• 1 tsp red wine vinegar

• 1 tsp caster sugar

• pinch of chilli flakes

• ½ small bunch of basil, torn, plus extra to serve

Directions

• STEP 1

Heat 175ml water in a saucepan until steaming, then add the butter. Remove from the heat and leave to cool until the mixture is just warm (it should not be hot). Combine the flour, yeast, sugar and 1 tsp salt in a large bowl or stand mixer. Add the cooled butter mixture, and mix to a soft dough using a wooden spoon or the mixer. Knead for 10 mins by hand (or 5 mins using a mixer) until the dough feels bouncy and smooth. Transfer to an oiled bowl and cover with a clean tea towel. Leave somewhere warm to rise for 1½-2 hrs, or until doubled in size. Alternatively, leave to prove in the fridge overnight.

• STEP 2

Oil and line a baking sheet with baking parchment. Knock the air out of the dough, then knead again for several minutes. Flatten a small piece of dough (about 20g) into a disc, and put a cube of the mozzarella and a pinch of the gruyère into the middle of the disc. Enclose the cheeses with the dough, then roll into a ball. Transfer to the prepared baking sheet. Repeat with the remaining cheese and dough, placing the dough balls ½cm apart on the baking sheet – they should be just touching after proving. Cover with a clean tea towel and leave somewhere warm to rise for 30 mins.

• STEP 3

Meanwhile, make the garlic butter. Melt the butter in a small pan over a low heat, then stir in the garlic and rosemary. Remove from the heat and set aside until needed. Heat the oven to 180C/160C fan/gas 4. Brush the risen dough balls with the garlic butter, then bake for 25-30 mins until the dough balls are cooked through and the middles are oozing.

• STEP 4

While the dough balls are baking, make the tomato sauce dip. Heat the oil in a saucepan and fry the garlic for 30 seconds. Tip in the passata, vinegar, sugar and chilli flakes, and simmer for 10 mins until thickened. Season to taste and stir in the basil. Brush the warm dough balls with any remaining garlic butter, then serve with the tomato sauce dip on the side for dunking.

Easy plum jam

Ingredients

- 2kg plums, stoned and roughly chopped

- 2kg white granulated sugar

- 2 tsp ground cinnamon

- 1 tbsp lemon juice

- 3 cinnamon sticks (optional)

- knob of butter

Directions

- STEP 1

Sterilise the jars and any other equipment before you start (see tip). Put a couple of saucers in the freezer, as you'll need these for testing whether the jam is ready later (or use a sugar thermometer). Put the plums in a preserving pan and add 200ml water. Bring to a simmer, and cook for about 10 mins until the plums are tender but not falling apart. Add the sugar, ground cinnamon and lemon juice, then let the sugar dissolve slowly, without boiling. This will take about 10 mins.

• STEP 2

Increase the heat and bring the jam to a full rolling boil. After about 5 mins, spoon a little jam onto a cold saucer. Wait a few seconds, then push the jam with your fingertip. If it wrinkles, the jam is ready. If not, cook for a few mins more and test again, with another cold saucer. If you have a sugar thermometer, it will read 105C when ready.

• STEP 3

Take the jam off the heat and add the cinnamon sticks (if using) and the knob of butter. The cinnamon will look pretty in the jars and the butter will disperse any scum. Let the jam cool for 15 mins, which will prevent the lumps of fruit sinking to the bottom of the jars. Ladle into hot jars, seal and leave to cool. Will keep for 1 year in a cool, dark place. Chill once opened.

Caramelised mushroom tartlets

Ingredients

• 2 tbsp olive oil

• 1 onion, chopped

• 1 tbsp golden caster sugar

• 250g chestnut mushrooms, cleaned and thinly sliced

• 1 garlic clove, crushed

• 3-4 tbsp thyme leaves, finely chopped

• butter, for spreading

• 12 slices of thin sliced white sandwich bread

• 100g grated gruyère or cheddar, for sprinkling

Directions

• STEP 1

Heat the oil in a generous frying pan, add the onion and fry over moderate heat for about 7 mins until soft and golden. Stir in the sugar and seasoning, turn up the heat and add the mushrooms. Sizzle for 5 mins until you have driven off any moisture and the mushrooms are golden. Stir in the garlic for a few further mins, until fragrant, then turn off the heat and stir in most of the thyme (save some for sprinkling). The mushroom mix can be chilled at this point.

• STEP 2

To make the tartlet bases, cut 7-8cm circles out of the bread using a cookie cutter or glass. Butter one side and stick buttered-side down into a 12-hole tartlet tin. Freeze any leftovers to make breadcrumbs.

• STEP 3

When ready to bake, heat oven to 220C/200 fan/gas 7. Divide the mushroom mixture between the tartlets and top with a sprinkle of cheese. Don't be too tidy about this – any cheese on the tin will form a lacy edge to the tartlets. Bake for 10-15 mins until golden and bubbling. Sprinkle over the reserved herbs and serve.

Ricotta and basil pizza

Ingredients

• 1 onion, finely chopped

• 2 yellow peppers, roughly chopped

• 1 tsp olive oil

• 2 x 400g/14oz cans chopped tomatoes

• 500g bag mixed grain or granary bread mix

• plain flour, for dusting

• 10 cherry tomatoes, halved or whole

• 250g tub ricotta

• a few basil leaves, to serve

Directions

• STEP 1

Heat oven to 220C/fan 200C/gas 6. Soften the onion and peppers in the oil in a large pan for a few mins.

Pour in the tomatoes, season, then simmer for 10 mins.

• STEP 2

Meanwhile, make up the bread mix according to pack instructions, then bring the dough together and knead a couple of times. Flour a large baking sheet and roll out the dough into a rectangle roughly 25 x 35cm. Bake for 5 mins on a shelf at the top of the oven until firm.

• STEP 3

Remove from the oven, spread with the sauce, add the cherry tomatoes, then dollop over spoonfuls of the ricotta. Bake for 10 mins more until the base is golden and crisp. Scatter with basil and serve straight away with a green salad.

DELIGHTFUL RECIPES FOR SOUP

Spicy Chickpea Soup with Kale

Ingredients

1 tablespoon olive oil

2 teaspoons cumin seeds

½ teaspoon red pepper flakes (Optional)

1 medium onion, minced

1 large carrot, peeled and diced

2 stalks celery, diced

3 cloves garlic, minced

4 cups chicken broth

1 (15 ounce) can chickpeas - rinsed, drained, and lightly smashed

1 small bunch kale, chopped

salt and ground black pepper to taste

½ cup finely chopped fresh parsley

1 tablespoon freshly grated Parmesan cheese, or to taste (Optional)

Directions

1. Heat olive oil over medium heat in a medium-sized pot until warm. Add cumin seeds and red pepper flakes; cook and stir until fragrant, about 30 seconds. Add onion, carrot, celery, and garlic; cook and stir until onion is softened and translucent, about 5 minutes. Stir in chicken broth, chickpeas, and kale.

2. Bring soup to a simmer and cook until kale is tender, 10 to 15 minutes. Season with salt and pepper; stir in parsley. Remove from heat; top with Parmesan cheese.

Turkish Red Lentil Soup with Mint

Ingredients

2 tablespoons olive oil

½ onion, diced

1 clove garlic, minced

¼ cup diced tomatoes, drained

5 cups chicken stock

½ cup red lentils

¼ cup fine bulgur

¼ cup rice

2 tablespoons tomato paste

1 tablespoon dried mint

1 teaspoon paprika

½ teaspoon cayenne pepper (Optional)

salt and ground black pepper to taste

Directions

1. Heat oil in a large pot over high heat. Add onion and sauté until beginning to soften, about 2 minutes. Stir in garlic and cook for 2 minutes. Add diced tomatoes and cook for 10 minutes.

2. Stir in chicken stock, lentils, bulgur, rice, tomato paste, mint, paprika, cayenne pepper, salt, and black pepper; bring to a boil. Reduce the heat to

medium-low and simmer until lentils and rice are tender, about 30 minutes.

3. Purée soup with an immersion blender until smooth.

Quinoa and Vegetable Soup

Ingredients

2 tablespoons olive oil

2 tablespoons butter

1 onion, chopped

½ cup diced carrot

½ cup chopped celery

1 clove garlic, minced

2 (32 ounce) cartons chicken broth

1 (28 ounce) can crushed tomatoes

2 tablespoons dried parsley

1 teaspoon dried basil

1 bay leaf

1 pinch dried thyme

2 cups shredded cabbage

1 (15 ounce) can light red kidney beans, drained

½ cup quinoa

½ cup grated Parmesan cheese (Optional)

Directions

1. Heat olive oil and butter in a large pot or Dutch oven over medium heat. Add onion, carrot, celery, and garlic; cook and stir until softened, 3

to 5 minutes. Stir in chicken broth, tomatoes, parsley, basil, bay leaf, and thyme; bring to a boil. Reduce heat and simmer until heated through, about 5 minutes.

2. Stir cabbage, kidney beans, and quinoa into the soup. Cover and simmer until quinoa is tender, 30 minutes. Garnish each serving with Parmesan cheese.

Roasted Red Bell Pepper Soup

Ingredients

3 red bell peppers

1 onion, chopped

1 tablespoon minced garlic

1 tablespoon olive oil

2 (15 ounce) cans cannellini beans, drained and rinsed

2 (14.5 ounce) cans chicken broth

salt and pepper to taste

Directions

1. Preheat oven to broil.
2. Place the bell peppers on a baking sheet and broil on the top rack of the oven, using tongs to turn them as each side blackens. Place the blackened peppers in a paper bag, close tightly and allow them to cool for 20 to 30 minutes. Then peel the skin off the peppers and discard the stem and all the seeds. Chop the peppers and set aside.
3. In a large pot over medium heat, saute the onion and garlic in the oil for 5 minutes, or until onion is translucent. Now add the chopped, roasted

red bell peppers and saute for 2 to 3 more minutes.

4. Next, add the chicken broth and the beans, stirring well. Using a blender, puree the soup in small batches and return to the pot over low heat for 5 minutes.

Instant Pot Lentil Soup

Ingredients

3 tablespoons olive oil

½ onion, finely diced

1 carrot, peeled and diced

1 stalk celery, diced

2 cloves garlic, minced

2 teaspoons ground cumin

½ teaspoon ground coriander

½ teaspoon ground turmeric

½ teaspoon salt

½ teaspoon ground white pepper

¼ teaspoon fennel seeds

⅛ teaspoon chile powder

1 tablespoon tomato paste

4 cups vegetable broth

3 cups water

1 ¼ cups green lentils

1 small yellow squash, diced (Optional)

1 cube vegetable bouillon

1 lemon, juiced

1 cup chopped kale, or to taste

Directions

1. Turn on a multi-functional pressure cooker
    (such as Instant Pot®) and select Saute function.
    Warm olive oil for 3 minutes. Add onion, carrot,
    celery, and garlic. Cook until onion is soft and
    translucent, 4 to 5 minutes. Season with cumin,
    coriander, turmeric, salt, white pepper, fennel,
    and chile powder. Cook for 2 more minutes. Stir
    in tomato paste.

2. Pour in broth and water. Stir in lentils and
    squash. Crumble bouillon cube over the top and
    mix well, scraping the bottom of the pan to
    remove any browned bits. Cancel Saute Mode.

3. Close and lock the lid. Select high pressure according to manufacturer's instructions; set timer for 8 minutes. Allow 10 to 15 minutes for pressure to build.

4. Release pressure using the natural-release method according to manufacturer's instructions for 10 minutes. Open valve to vent remaining steam, about 5 minutes. Unlock and remove the lid.

5. Mix in lemon juice and toss kale leaves just on top of the soup. Replace lid and allow kale to steam for about 5 minutes. Remove lid and adjust seasonings, if desired, before serving.

Garden Gazpacho

Ingredients

1 large English cucumber - halved, seeded, and chopped

2 red bell peppers, seeded and chopped

½ cup chopped red onion

2 stalks celery, chopped

5 plum tomatoes, quartered and seeded

2 cloves garlic, or more to taste

3 cups low-sodium tomato juice

¼ cup white wine vinegar

¼ cup extra-virgin olive oil

1 teaspoon freshly ground black pepper

1 teaspoon sea salt

1 teaspoon dried basil

1 teaspoon dried parsley

½ teaspoon red pepper flakes, or more to taste (Optional)

Directions

1. Place cucumber in a food processor; pulse 5 to 6 times to chop into very small pieces. Transfer to a large bowl. Repeat with red bell peppers, red onion, and celery, pulsing each into very small pieces in the food processor and transferring to the bowl.

2. Combine plum tomatoes and garlic in the food processor; pulse until finely diced. Pour over cucumber mixture in the bowl.

3. Pour tomato juice, white wine vinegar, and olive oil over tomato and cucumber mixture in the bowl. Add sea salt, black pepper, basil, parsley, and red pepper flakes; stir well.

4. Chill until flavors combine and deepen, about 2 hours.

Easy Curried Cauliflower Soup

Ingredients

1 tablespoon olive oil, or as needed

½ onion, sliced, or to taste

3 carrots, cut into 1/2-inch slices

½ red bell pepper, sliced

3 cloves garlic, peeled, or more to taste

1 head cauliflower, chopped

1 (32 fluid ounce) container chicken stock, or as needed

2 tablespoons yellow curry powder

1 tablespoon butter

4 dashes hot sauce (such as Tapatio®), or more to taste

salt and ground black pepper to taste

Directions

1. Heat olive oil in a large pot over medium heat; cook and stir onion, carrots, red bell pepper, and garlic until tender and softened, 5 to 10 minutes. Add cauliflower to vegetable mixture and pour in chicken broth; bring to a boil. Cook soup until cauliflower is tender, about 10 minutes.

2. Remove pot from heat and blend soup using a hand blender until smooth.

3. Place pot over low heat and add curry powder, butter, hot sauce, salt, and pepper to soup;

simmer until flavors have blended, about 15 minutes more.

Cold-Busting Ginger Chicken Noodle Soup

Ingredients

1 ½ tablespoons olive oil

3 large chicken breasts

1 large onion, diced

3 cloves garlic, crushed

13 cups water

2 cups white wine

¾ cup fresh lemon juice

1 (4 inch) piece fresh ginger, peeled and thinly sliced

1 tablespoon white sugar

4 cubes chicken bouillon

3 bay leaves

7 whole black peppercorns

¾ cup peeled and sliced carrots

2 stalks celery, diced

1 kohlrabi bulb, peeled and diced

2 ½ tablespoons fresh rosemary

2 tablespoons fresh thyme

1 (8 ounce) package egg noodles

1 large clove garlic, minced

1 tablespoon grated ginger

1 teaspoon salt, or to taste

½ cup chopped fresh parsley

Directions

1. Heat olive oil in a large pot over medium heat. Add chicken, onion, and crushed garlic cloves; cook until chicken is browned and onion starts to turn translucent, about 5 minutes. Pour water, wine, and lemon juice over chicken mixture; stir in sliced ginger, sugar, bouillon cubes, bay leaves, and peppercorns. Bring to a simmer, then reduce the heat to medium-low and cook for 45 minutes.

2. Remove and discard garlic cloves. Transfer chicken to a cutting board and chop into bite-size pieces.

3. Add carrots, celery, kohlrabi, rosemary, and thyme to the pot. Reduce the heat to low and cook until vegetables begin to soften, about 20 minutes.

4. Bring soup to a boil. Return chopped chicken to the pot along with egg noodles, minced garlic, and grated ginger. Remove from the heat and let sit until noodles have softened, about 10 minutes. Season with salt and garnish with parsley.

Spicy Lime Avocado Soup

Ingredients

2 skinless, boneless chicken breasts

1 tablespoon olive oil

1 large white onion, chopped, divided

1 cup chopped cilantro, divided

2 jalapeño peppers, halved and thinly sliced

3 limes, juiced

3 cloves garlic, minced

4 cups water

2 tablespoons reduced-sodium chicken bouillon powder

3 large firm, ripe avocados, cut into chunks

¼ cup crumbled queso fresco, or to taste

Directions

1. Bring a small pot of water to a boil. Add chicken; boil until an instant-read thermometer inserted into the center reads at least 165 degrees F (74 degrees C), about 7 minutes. Drain.

2. Run cool water over chicken to speed cooling process. Shred or finely slice chicken.

3. Heat olive oil in a large pot over medium heat. Add 1/2 of the onion, 1/2 cup cilantro, jalapeño peppers, lime juice, and garlic; cook until onion is slightly greenish in color, about 5 minutes.

4. Combine 4 cups water and bouillon powder in a small bowl; pour into the pot. Cook until just heated through, about 5 minutes. Stir in chicken.

5. Ladle soup into four bowls. Top with remaining avocado, onion, cilantro, and queso fresco.

Strawberry Gazpacho

Ingredients

3 pints hulled strawberries

½ cucumber - peeled, seeded, and chopped

½ onion, chopped

¼ cup chopped fresh cilantro

¼ cup chopped fresh parsley

1 pint hulled strawberries, chopped

½ cucumber - peeled, seeded, and chopped

½ onion, chopped

¼ cup chopped fresh cilantro

¼ cup chopped fresh parsley

1 bunch green onions, minced

1 jalapeno pepper, seeded and minced

⅓ cup red wine vinegar

3 tablespoons fresh lemon juice

2 tablespoons olive oil

1 ½ teaspoons salt

2 cloves garlic, minced

1 teaspoon dried tarragon

1 teaspoon dried basil

¼ teaspoon hot pepper sauce

⅛ teaspoon ground black pepper

1 large avocado - peeled, pitted, and cubed

Directions

1. Blend 3 pints strawberries, 1/2 the cucumber, 1/2 the onion, 1/4 cup cilantro, and 1/4 cup parsley in a blender on high speed until pureed, about 30 seconds. Pour the pureed mixture into a large bowl.

2. Stir 1 pint strawberries, 1/2 the cucumber, 1/2 the onion, 1/4 cup cilantro, 1/4 cup parsley, green onions, jalapeno pepper, red wine vinegar, lemon juice, olive oil, salt, garlic, tarragon, basil, hot pepper sauce, and black pepper into the pureed strawberry mixture. Spread avocado cubes over the top of the gazpacho.

3. Cover the bowl and chill gazpacho thoroughly, at least 2 hours, before serving.

Dairy-Free Creamy Broccoli Soup

Ingredients

1 tablespoon olive oil

1 large yellow onion, coarsely chopped

3 large cloves garlic, coarsely chopped

3 broccoli stalks, coarsely chopped

2 broccoli florets and stalks, coarsely chopped

2 large potatoes, peeled and coarsely chopped

⅓ celery root, coarsely chopped

4 cups low-sodium chicken stock

Directions

1. Heat olive oil in a saucepan over medium-low heat. Add onion and garlic; cook and stir until translucent, 10 to 15 minutes. Add broccoli stalks, potatoes, broccoli florets, and celery root; toss until coated in oil. Cover vegetables with chicken stock; bring to a boil.

2. Reduce heat and simmer, stirring occasionally, until vegetables are easily pierced with a fork, 20 to 25 minutes. Remove soup from heat.

3. Fill a blender no more than halfway with liquid and vegetables. Cover and hold lid down; pulse

a few times before increasing blender to maximum speed. Puree until soup is light green and creamy, 45 seconds to 1 minute. Repeat with remaining soup, working in batches.

Creamy Butternut Squash Soup with Fresh Ginger and Quinoa

Ingredients

1 tablespoon butter

1 tablespoon olive oil

1 onion, chopped

4 cups chicken broth

1 butternut squash - peeled, seeded, and cubed

1 (1 inch) piece fresh ginger, peeled and grated

1 teaspoon ground cumin

salt and ground black pepper to taste

2 cups water

1 cup quinoa

1 tablespoon butter

Directions

1. Heat 1 tablespoon butter and olive oil together in a skillet over medium heat; cook and stir onion until softened, 5 to 10 minutes. Add chicken broth, butternut squash, ginger, and cumin to onion and simmer over medium heat until squash is very soft, about 20 minutes.

2. Pour squash mixture into a blender no more than half full. Cover and hold lid down; pulse a few times before leaving on to blend. Puree in

batches until smooth. Season soup with salt and pepper.

3. Bring salted water and quinoa to a boil in a saucepan. Reduce heat to medium-low, cover, and simmer until quinoa is tender and water has been absorbed, 15 to 20 minutes. Stir 1 tablespoon butter into cooked quinoa and season with salt. Spoon quinoa into soup.

Sweet Potato and Kale Soup

Ingredients

2 tablespoons olive oil

1 onion, diced

2 cloves garlic, minced

1 teaspoon ground turmeric

1 teaspoon salt

¾ teaspoon curry powder

¾ teaspoon ground coriander

1 pound sweet potatoes, peeled and cut into 1/2-inch
cubes

4 cups vegetable broth

4 cups chopped kale

1 (15.5 ounce) can chickpeas, drained

1 cup canned coconut milk

Directions

1. Heat oil in a large stockpot over medium-high
    heat. Add onion and garlic and saute for 2
    minutes. Stir in turmeric, coriander, curry

powder, and coriander. Add sweet potatoes; saute for 2 to 3 minutes, stirring frequently.

2. Pour in broth and bring to a simmer. Cover and simmer until sweet potatoes have just begun to soften, 8 to 10 minutes. Stir in kale and chick peas; simmer for 5 minutes more. Stir in coconut milk and adjust salt to taste.

Simple Roasted Tomato Soup

Ingredients

3 pounds Roma (plum) tomatoes, quartered

1 yellow onion, halved and quartered

½ cup coarsely chopped red bell pepper

3 tablespoons olive oil

1 ½ teaspoons salt

1 ½ teaspoons ground black pepper

3 cloves garlic, halved

5 cups low-sodium chicken broth

2 tablespoons chopped fresh basil

2 tablespoons chopped fresh parsley

Directions

1. Preheat the oven to 400 degrees F (200 degrees C). Line two 10x15-inch baking pans with parchment paper.
2. Arrange tomatoes, onion, and bell pepper in a single layer on the prepared baking pans. Drizzle with oil and sprinkle with salt and pepper.
3. Roast in the preheated oven for 30 minutes. Add garlic; continue roasting until mixture is tender, about 15 minutes more.

4. Bring broth to a boil in a large pot over high heat. Reduce heat and simmer, covered.

5. Meanwhile, put 1/2 of the tomato mixture in a blender. Cover and pulse 3 times, then blend until smooth, adding hot broth as needed. Pour into the pot with broth. Repeat with remaining tomato mixture, then stir into the pot until combined.

6. Simmer soup to heat through, about 5 minutes. Stir in basil and parsley.

5

TO WRAP THINGS UP!

One of your greatest challenges of living with vasculitis may be coping with side effects of your medication. The following suggestions may help:

Understand your condition: Learn everything you can about vasculitis and its treatment. Know the possible side effects of the drugs you take, and tell your doctor about any changes in your health.

Follow your treatment plan: Your treatment plan may include seeing your doctor regularly, undergoing more tests and checking your blood pressure.

Choose a healthy diet: Eating well can help prevent potential problems that can result from your medications, such as thinning bones, high blood pressure and diabetes. Choose a diet that emphasizes fresh fruits and vegetables, whole grains, low-fat dairy products, and lean meats and fish. If you're taking a corticosteroid drug, ask your doctor if you need to take a vitamin D or calcium supplement.

Get routine vaccinations: Keeping up to date on vaccinations, such as for the flu and pneumonia, can help prevent problems that can result from your medications, such as infection. Talk to your doctor about vaccinations.

Exercise most days of the week: Regular aerobic exercise, such as walking, can help prevent bone loss, high blood pressure and diabetes that can be associated with taking corticosteroids. It also benefits your heart and lungs. In addition, many people find that exercise improves their mood and overall sense of well-being. If you're not used to exercising, start out slowly and build up gradually. Your doctor can help you plan an exercise program that's right for you.

Maintain a strong support system: Family and friends can help you as you cope with this condition. If you think it would be helpful to talk with other people who are living with vasculitis, ask a member of your health care team about connecting with a support group.